Sensei Self Development

Mental Health Chronicles Series

Building Resilience and Coping Strategies

Sensei Paul David

Copyright Page

Sensei Self Development -
Building Resilience and Coping Strategies,
by Sensei Paul David

Copyright © 2024

All rights reserved.

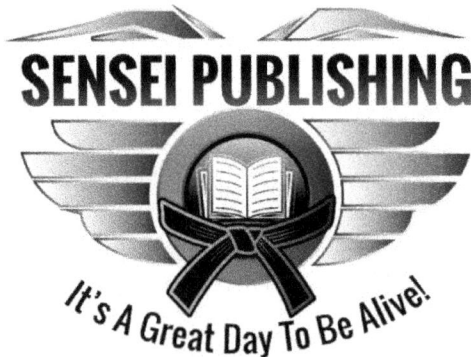

www.senseipublishing.com

@senseipublishing
#senseipublishing

Get/Share Your FREE SSD Mental Health Chronicles at
www.senseiselfdevelopment.care

or

CLICK HERE

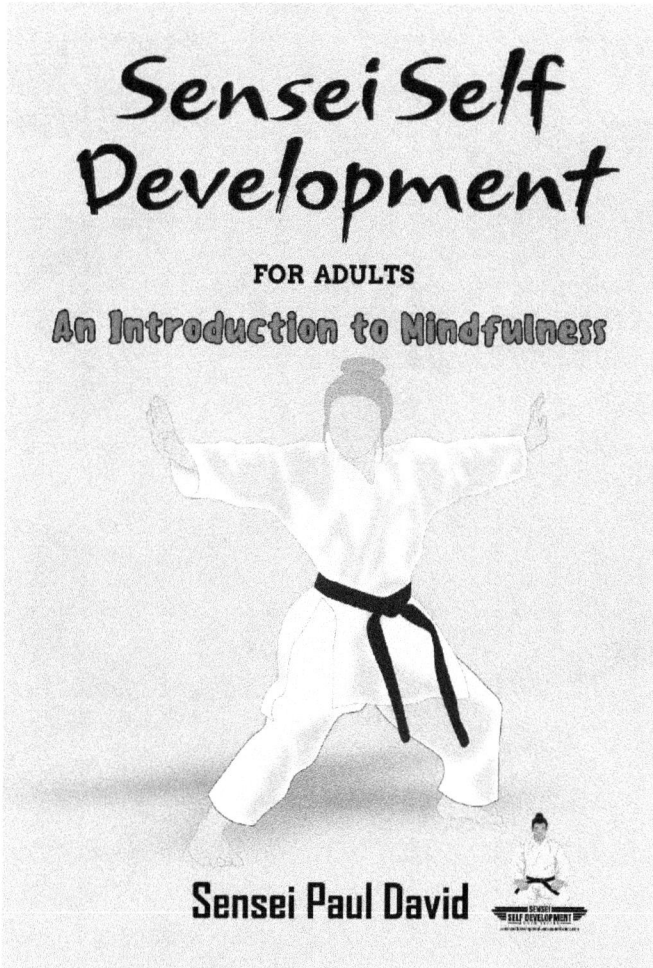

Check Out The SSD Chronicles
Series CLICK HERE

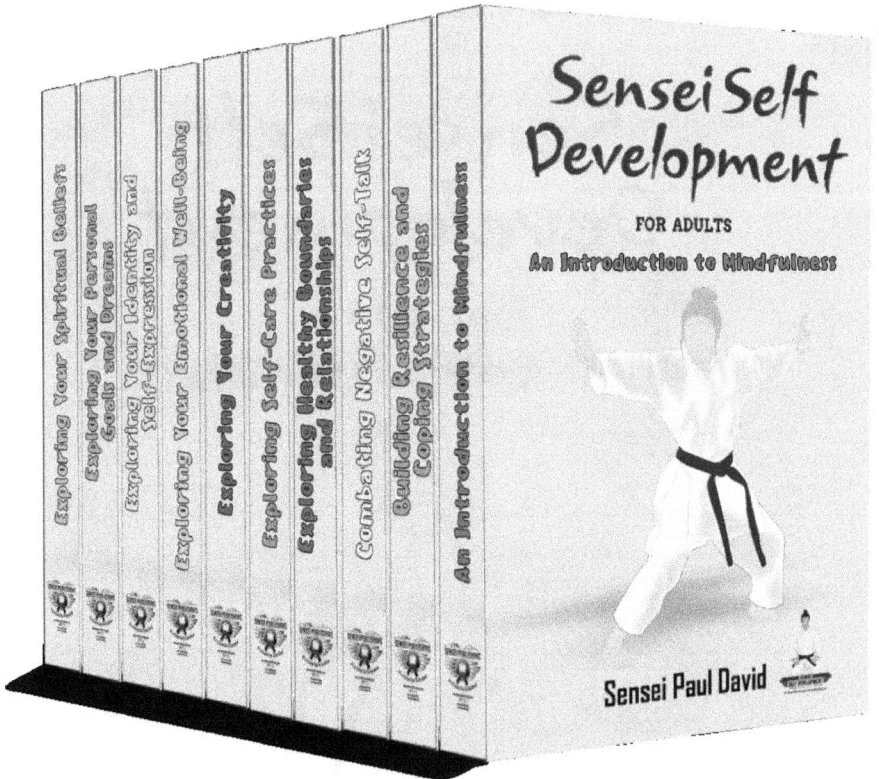

Exploring Your Spiritual Beliefs

Exploring Your Personal Goals and Dreams

Exploring Your Identity and Self-Expression

Exploring Your Emotional Well-Being

Exploring Your Creativity

Exploring Self-Care Practices

Exploring Healthy Boundaries and Relationships

Combatting Negative Self-Talk

Building Resilience and Coping Strategies

An Introduction to Mindfulness

Sensei Self Development

FOR ADULTS

An Introduction to Mindfulness

Sensei Paul David

Dedication

To those who courageously take action towards self-improvement - you are helping to evolve the world for generations to come.

- It's a great day to be alive!

If Found Please Contact:

_____

Reward If Found:

_____

MY
COMMITMENT

I, _____

commit to writing This Sensei Self Development Journal for at least 10 days in a row, starting: _____

Writing this journal is valuable to me because:

_____

_____

_____

_____

_____

_____

If I finish a minimum of 10 consecutive days of writing in this journal, I will reward myself by:

_____

_____

_____

_____

_____

_____

If I don't finish 10 days of writing this journal, I will promise to:

_____

_____

_____

_____

_____

I will do the following things to ensure that I write in my Sensei Self Development Journal every day:

_____

_____

_____

_____

_____

Get/Share Your FREE All-Ages Mental Health eBook Now at

www.senseiselfdevelopment.com

Or CLICK HERE

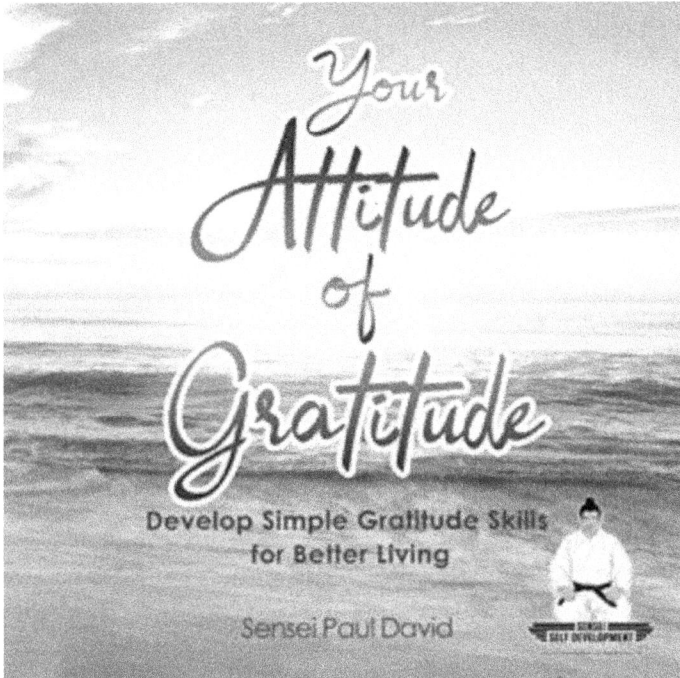

senseiselfdevelopment.com

Check Out Another Book In The SSD BOOK SERIES:

senseipublishing.com/SSD_SERIES

CLICK HERE

SENSEI
SELF DEVELOPMENT
BOOKS SERIES

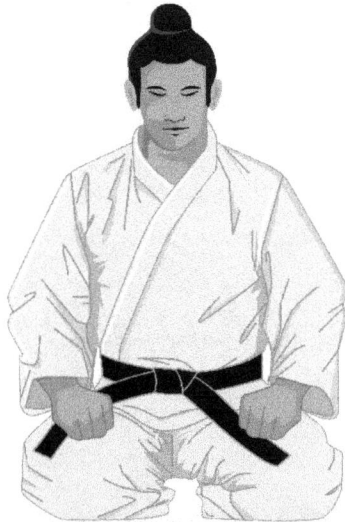

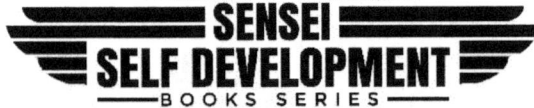

senseiselfdevelopment.senseipublishing.com

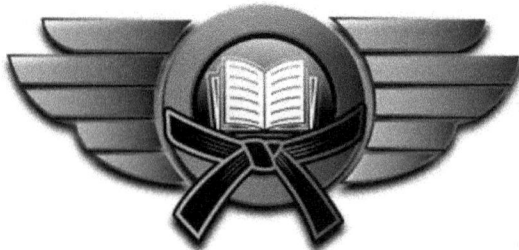

Join Our Publishing Journey!

If you would like to receive FUTURE FREE BOOKS and get to know us better, please click www.senseipublishing.com and join our newsletter by entering your email address in the pop-up box.

Follow Our Blog: senseipauldavid.ca

Follow/Like/Subscribe: Facebook, Instagram, YouTube: @senseipublishing

Scan the QR Code with your phone or tablet

to follow us on social media: Like / Subscribe / Follow

A Message From The Author:
Sensei Paul David

Dear Reader,

Welcome to the world of mental health journaling – a sacred space for self-reflection, growth, and healing. Within these pages, you hold the power to uplift your spirit, invigorate your mind, and nourish your goals.

In a world that often moves at blink-and-you'll-miss-it speed, it's crucial to make time for self-care and self-discovery.

Anxiety, stress, and emotional turbulence may have clouded your mind, making it difficult to find clarity and peace within. But fear not! Together, we will navigate the labyrinth of emotions, and experiences, helping to simplify the path to mental well-being.

This journal is not merely a bunch of blank pages awaiting your words. It is your compassionate companion, offering solace and understanding during your unique journey. Here, you are free to unburden yourself, celebrate small and large victories, and confront the challenges that may still linger.

Within the sheltered realm of these pages, there is no judgment, no expectation, and no pressure. Your unique experience and perspective hold immeasurable worth, and your voice deserves to be heard. Whether you choose to fill the lines with eloquence or simply scribble fragments of your thoughts, please remember each entry is a valuable contribution to your growth.

In this sacred space, you are challenged to take off the mask we so often wear in the outside world. It is here that you can be raw, vulnerable, and authentic – allowing your true self to be seen and embraced without reservation. By giving yourself permission to explore the depths of your emotions and confront the shadows that may lurk within, you will discover profound insights and find the healing you seek over time.

As you embark on this journaling journey, I encourage you to embrace the process itself rather than fixate solely on the outcome. Remember, it is not about reaching a certain destination or ticking off boxes on a list of accomplishments. Rather, it is about cultivating self-awareness, fostering self-compassion, and nurturing a sense of curiosity about the intricate workings of your intelligently beautiful mind.

In the quiet moments of reflection, let your pen become a bridge between your inner world and the possibilities that lie ahead. Create a sanctuary for your thoughts, fears, triumphs, and dreams. As you pour your heart onto these pages, allow your words to be a living testament to courage, resilience, and an unwavering commitment to your own well-being.

I am honored to be a part of your journey, and I believe in your ability to navigate the twists and turns with grace and resilience. Remember, you are not alone in this – countless others have walked similar paths, faced similar challenges, and emerged stronger and wiser on the other side. You have the power to reclaim all of your untapped joy, cultivate a positive mindset that serves you, and foster a deep sense of self-love and peaceful confident. – And it will take a worth effort and time.

So, open the first page of this journal with hope, curiosity, and an open heart and open mind. Embrace the transformative power of self-reflection, and allow it to guide you towards a life of greater fulfilment and peace. Each journaling session is an opportunity to not only connect with yourself but also to rekindle the light within that sometimes flickers but never extinguishes.

Remember, the pages you are about to fill are not just a record of your journey but also a testament to your strength, resilience, and indomitable spirit. Cherish this space, invest in yourself, and let your words be an ode to the magnificent journey of becoming whole.

With great respect for your decision to evolve,

Paul

MY CONVICTION

Please circle your answers below

I am DECIDING to be patient with myself and this PROCESS each time I journal toward my improved state of mental well-being

YES   NO

"The present moment is filled with joy and happiness. If you are attentive, you will see it."

Thich Nhat Hanh

Introduction

What Resilience Is

Resilience is a coping skill. It is the practical ability to recover quickly from difficulties. It's like having a mental and emotional toolkit that helps you bounce back from setbacks. For instance, if you lose your job, resilience is what helps you cope with the initial shock and stress, and then motivates you to update your resume and start applying for new positions, rather than getting stuck in despair.

It's about facing life's problems head-on, rather than avoiding them. Imagine you have a leak in your roof. Resilience is grabbing a bucket to catch the water, calling a repair service, and perhaps figuring out a temporary fix, instead of just hoping the leak will stop on its own.

Resilience doesn't mean you don't feel upset, scared, or angry about life's challenges. It's perfectly normal to have these feelings. What makes you resilient is your ability to experience these emotions and then find a way to move forward, instead of being paralyzed by them.

In daily life, resilience can show up in small ways. It's about how you handle a stressful day at work or how you manage to keep going even when you're juggling multiple responsibilities and everything feels overwhelming.

The good news is resilience can be built and strengthened over time, much like a muscle. It's developed through practices like setting realistic goals, connecting with others for support, and learning to reframe negative thoughts into more positive, or at least neutral, ones.

All in all, resilience is a practical, everyday skill that helps you deal with life's challenges in a healthy, constructive way. It's not about avoiding problems, but about having the tools and mindset to face them effectively.

What Resilience Isn't

Resilience is not about never facing challenges or feeling distressed. It doesn't mean you glide through life without facing any problems. Everyone encounters challenges; resilience is about how you deal with them.

Resilience should not be seen as a personality trait exclusive to some. Rather, it's about adopting certain behaviors, ways of thinking, and actions that can be learned and cultivated by anyone. This universality of resilience is supported by research, as seen in widespread resilient responses to events like the September 11, 2001, terrorist attacks, where many sought to rebuild their lives in the aftermath of tragedy.

Building resilience is similar to strengthening a muscle; it requires time and deliberate effort. By focusing on key areas – forming strong connections, maintaining wellness, practicing healthy thinking, and finding meaning – you can enhance your ability to endure and grow from challenging and traumatic experiences.

Adopting these strategies can bolster your resilience, helping you not just to survive difficult times but to thrive through them.

Characteristics of Highly Resilient Individuals

Resilient individuals often stand out for their unique approach to life's challenges. Steven M. Southwick, a renowned expert in psychiatry and resilience at Yale University School of Medicine, highlights several key characteristics that define these resilient people:

1. Optimism Paired with Realism: They tend to see the glass half full, but without losing sight of reality. This positive outlook doesn't ignore the negatives; rather, it seeks to find the silver lining in difficult situations.

2. Strong Moral Compass: Resilient people often have a clear sense of right and wrong, which acts as a guiding force in their decision-making process.

3. Faith in Something Greater: Many find strength in religious or spiritual beliefs. This sense of being part of something bigger than themselves, coupled with the support of a like-minded community, greatly bolsters their resilience.

4. Altruism: There's a noticeable concern for others and a tendency towards selflessness. They are often deeply involved in causes that matter to them, providing a sense of fulfillment and purpose.

5. Acceptance and Adaptability: What sets resilient individuals apart is their ability to accept what can't be changed and pivot their focus to what they can influence. They are adept at finding meaningful opportunities in challenging circumstances.

6. Purpose-Driven Life: A clear mission or purpose in life gives them a sense of direction, courage, and strength.

7. Robust Social Networks: Resilient people often have a strong circle of friends and family who they rely on, and they reciprocate that support.

These traits not only help them navigate through life's ups and downs but also serve as a roadmap for anyone looking to strengthen their own resilience.

How to Become More Resilient

Become an optimist

Studies have shown that optimistic people tend to cope better with stress, have stronger immune systems, and even enjoy longer lifespans. This is because optimism helps us approach problems with a mindset that is geared toward finding solutions and learning from experiences, rather than being overwhelmed by them.

The best way to become more optimistic is to think like an optimist.

Optimism is deeply rooted in the stories we tell ourselves when faced with life's ups and downs. This narrative style, known as our "explanatory style," can significantly influence how we perceive and respond to challenges. It revolves around three key aspects: permanence, pervasiveness, and personalization, commonly referred to as the 3 P's.

Permanence: When something goes wrong, an optimist sees it as a temporary obstacle. They think, "This is just a hiccup, it'll pass." On the contrary, a pessimist might view the same situation as a permanent fixture in their life, thinking, "This is always going to be a problem for me."

Pervasiveness: Optimists see problems as specific to a situation and not reflective of their entire life. They remind themselves, "This is just one aspect; it doesn't change all the good things I have going on." Pessimists, however, might see an issue as all-encompassing, believing, "This is going to ruin everything."

Personalization: When it comes to personalization, optimists don't internalize the blame. They understand that external factors often play a role, thinking, "This happened because of something outside my control." Pessimists, in contrast, often take setbacks personally: "It's all my fault."

Understanding these differences in perspective is crucial. For pessimists, challenges can feel like insurmountable walls, leading to feelings of helplessness and sometimes depression. Optimists, however, view these challenges as temporary and specific hurdles, maintaining a sense of hope and resilience.

Fortunately, our explanatory style isn't set in stone. We can learn to shift from a pessimistic to an optimistic viewpoint by consciously reframing our thoughts. When faced with adversity, instead of automatically thinking, "This always happens to me," we can remind ourselves, "This is a one-time event." We can train ourselves to see problems as specific and not indicative of our entire lives.

Adopting a more optimistic explanatory style involves a deliberate effort to change our internal narrative.

Remember the three Ps: Permanence, Pervasiveness, and personalization. And think more like an optimist would.

Practice Acceptance

Practicing acceptance means recognizing the reality of a situation and finding ways to live with it, rather than against it. For example, if you're stuck in traffic and late for an appointment, acceptance is understanding that there's nothing you can do to change the traffic situation. Instead of stewing in frustration, you might turn on some music or an audiobook, making the most of the time you have in the car.

This practice can be particularly helpful for dealing with minor annoyances. Say your partner constantly forgets to turn off the lights, which annoys you. Acceptance involves recognizing this isn't a major flaw but a human quirk. Instead of letting it become a source of constant irritation, you might gently remind them or find humor in their forgetfulness. This shift in perspective reduces stress and preserves peace at home.

For those who live alone, acceptance could involve coming to terms with feelings of loneliness. Rather than dwelling on the solitude, you might see it as an opportunity to pick up new hobbies or reconnect with old friends over the phone.

The process of acceptance involves first acknowledging that a situation is stressful or less than ideal. Then, it's about shifting focus to the aspects you can control or influence. For instance, if you're overwhelmed with a busy schedule, acceptance is recognizing that you can't change the number of hours in a day, but you can prioritize tasks and perhaps say no to new commitments. It's about making peace with the elements you can't change and taking action on the ones you can.

Take Action

When dealing with a loss or a challenging situation, it's common to experience ambivalence, especially when things aren't clear-cut. You might find yourself feeling uncertain about how to feel or what steps to take next. This mix of conflicting emotions and thoughts is a normal part of processing complex situations.

Waiting for complete clarity is never the best approach. The search for absolute certainty can lead to hesitation, which often results in inaction. When you're stuck in a state of indecision, life can feel like it's on pause. This can add to the stress and uncertainty of the situation.

Instead, it's often more beneficial to make decisions, even if they're not perfect. Taking action, even with less-than-ideal choices, can help move you forward and out of the state of limbo. Making a decision, even a small one, can provide a sense of control and progress. It's about accepting that in complex and uncertain situations, perfect clarity might be unattainable, and that's okay.

Use Premortem

Resilience does not mean you only prepare psychologically. It also means you prepare physically. Someone who is always prepared is a more resilient individual because they can deal with bad situations effectively.

Think of a premortem as a mental rehearsal for what could go wrong in any situation you're planning. For instance, you're organizing a family picnic. A premortem approach would have you imagine it's the day of the picnic, and everything that could go wrong, did go wrong. It rained, the food wasn't enough, someone forgot the sunscreen, and the spot you chose was too crowded.

In this imagined scenario, you identify all these potential problems before they happen. Then, you plan accordingly: check the weather forecast and have a backup indoor location, prepare extra food, make a checklist for essentials like sunscreen, and scout for alternative spots.

So, if any one of these bad situations shows its ugly head, you are prepared to deal with it. That's resilience.

Self Compassion

Self-compassion is about treating ourselves with the same kindness and understanding we would offer a good friend. It means acknowledging our own suffering and approaching it with warmth, without judgment. Research has shown that engaging in practices of self-compassion can lead to increased mindfulness and life satisfaction, while reducing feelings of depression, anxiety, and stress. These benefits can last for an extended period, even up to a year.

A practical tool for self-compassion is the "Self-Compassion Break," which can be particularly helpful when you're feeling overwhelmed. It consists of three steps that align with the principles of self-compassion:

1. **Mindfulness:** Recognize and acknowledge your feelings without judgment. You might say to yourself, "This is a moment of suffering," "This hurts," or "I'm feeling stressed."

2. **Common Humanity:** Remind yourself that you're not alone in these feelings. Everyone goes through tough times. You could tell yourself, "Suffering is part of life," or "We all struggle in our lives."

3. **Self-Kindness:** Offer yourself kindness and understanding. Placing your hands on your heart, say something like, "May I be compassionate to myself," "May I accept myself as I am," or "May I be patient with myself."

For those who find it hard to be kind to themselves, the exercise "How Would You

Treat a Friend?" can be eye-opening. It involves comparing how you react to your own struggles versus how you would respond to a friend's. This comparison often reveals a harsher attitude towards oneself, prompting valuable reflections on why this is and how things might change if you were gentler with yourself.

Another helpful practice is writing a "Self-Compassionate Letter." Spend 15 minutes writing to yourself about a specific struggle you feel ashamed of, such as being shy or not spending enough time with your children. In the letter, remind yourself that everyone has struggles and consider constructive ways to address this in the future. This exercise helps to solidify a more compassionate and understanding voice towards yourself.

Have Resilient Role Models

Having role models of resilience is a powerful way to foster your own resilience. This involves looking up to individuals who have demonstrated perseverance in overcoming challenges, including traumatic experiences. Your role models could be anyone who inspires you with their strength and tenacity – it could be a family member, a friend, a teacher, a pastor, or a community leader. The key is their ability to face and surmount adversity.

You don't necessarily need to have a personal relationship with these individuals to draw inspiration from their stories. For example, someone might find inspiration in historical figures like Franklin Delano Roosevelt. They might never have met him, but learning about how he overcame the challenges of polio and went on to lead a country can be incredibly motivating and instructive.

Identifying and learning from the resilience of others can provide valuable lessons in perseverance and strength, offering a blueprint for handling our own challenges more effectively. These role models serve as a reminder of the human capacity to overcome adversity, inspiring us to cultivate similar qualities in our own lives.

Build and Maintain Connection

In tough times, it's natural to want to retreat into solitude, driven by feelings like shame, fear of judgment, or not wanting to burden others. However, it's crucial to maintain connection with people. Studies indicate that the absence of social support post-trauma can increase the risk of developing post-traumatic stress disorder.

Remember avoiding contact with friends and family means they can't offer support.

When facing overwhelming challenges, reach out for support. This could be by sharing your experiences with someone who listens without judgment. Let them know if you just need a listening ear. Or, seek specific help, like advice or assistance with tasks. Recognize that asking for help, far from being a weakness, demonstrates courage.

To foster connections and support, consider these strategies: invite someone to exercise or walk with you, regularly contact loved ones, engage in playful activities with friends, join groups with shared interests, or volunteer to help others.

Moreover, according to research, having good relationships – family, friends, acquaintances, and so on – is the single best thing for an individual's overall well-being. So, relationships are important not just important for resilience, or to protect yourself from adversity, but to actually live a good life itself. For most of us, a good life is not possible if we have no one to share it with.

Practice Positive Reappraisal

Positive reappraisal involves looking at a challenging situation and finding a way to see it in a more positive light. For example, during the pandemic, many people found themselves missing activities like concerts or visiting friends. However, by using positive reappraisal, they shifted their focus to the new opportunities the situation presented: more time for reading, cooking, or reconnecting with distant friends through Zoom.

So, try to look at the bright side of any situation. And there is always a bright side, even in death and destruction. Remember that. The event might not be bright in itself but at least it revealed something to you.

Label Your Emotions

Many people attempt to manage uncomfortable emotions by suppressing them, believing it grants control. However, this approach, especially when habitual, can hinder resilience against life's challenges. A study involving several volunteers found that people who consistently tried to avoid or control their emotions experienced less enjoyment in daily activities and felt more negative emotions. Constantly dodging emotions or attempting to suppress them can prevent you from being present and fully engaging in daily life.

While occasional avoidance can be a valid emotional regulation strategy, relying on it can be detrimental. Instead, develop a more constructive relationship with your emotions. When confronted with difficult emotions, rather than pushing them away, identify and name them specifically. Rather than saying "I feel bad," pinpoint the exact feeling, like "I'm disappointed" or "I'm frustrated." Accurately labeling emotions can lessen their intensity. Explore these emotions with curiosity. Consider what the emotion is communicating and its underlying purpose. For instance, feeling disappointed due to a lie may highlight the importance of honesty to you. Every emotion, even the challenging ones, serves a purpose and provides valuable insights into your values and potential areas for change in your life.

Psychological Flexibility

The concept of resilience is often misunderstood as simply being tough or unyielding in the face of adversity. However, resilience is more about being psychologically flexible and adaptable, because the same approach may not work for every challenge you face.

Let's consider a concrete example: losing your job during a challenging time. This event is likely to trigger a range of emotions like sadness, fear, or even panic.

Initially, calming strategies might be most effective. This could include activities that provide a temporary distraction from the immediate stress, such as engaging in a hobby or watching a movie. Alternatively, expressing your feelings to a trusted friend or family member can also be a helpful initial response, providing emotional release and perspective.

However, resilience isn't just about initial coping; it's also about switching your strategies over time. As you move beyond the initial shock of job loss, it becomes important to shift gears. This is where strategies like reappraisal come into play. Reappraisal involves looking at the situation in a new light. For example, you might start to see the job loss as an opportunity to explore new career paths or to develop skills that you wouldn't have had the time or motivation to focus on previously.

The key is to have a diverse set of coping strategies and to know when to use which strategy. In some cases, distraction might be a temporary solution to help you get through an immediate crisis, but it's not a long-term strategy. If used excessively, it could prevent you from addressing the underlying issues or emotions. Reappraisal, on the other hand, is particularly effective in situations that are out of your control. It allows you to find a sense of agency and possibility in circumstances that initially seem bleak or overwhelming.

Understanding and adapting these strategies requires self-awareness. It's important to recognize how specific circumstances impact you emotionally and mentally. This awareness enables you to select the most appropriate coping mechanism for each situation. For instance, in a situation where you have some control, problem-solving strategies might be more effective. In contrast, in situations where you have little control, acceptance and emotional support might be more beneficial.

In essence, resilience is about flexibility and creativity in coping. It's a dynamic process that involves not just enduring hardships but also learning from them and growing. By effectively adapting your coping strategies to fit specific situations, you enhance your ability to overcome adversity and emerge stronger and more resourceful.

Use Your Character Strength

Another crucial element in building resilience is leveraging your psychological strengths. These positive qualities, such as optimism, hope, courage, and humor, support your well-being and adaptability. Engaging in strengths-based practices, like using personal strengths in everyday life or performing acts of kindness, has been shown to enhance wellbeing.

To find out what virtues you have, take a survey online, the VIA Character Strengths Survey. It was developed by the father of positive psychology and has been proven to be very effective.

Find Meaning

Having meaning in life is like having a personal anchor. It gives you stability and a reason to hold on, especially when things get tough. This could be anything that's important to you – your family, a hobby, a dream, or a cause you believe in.

Resilience is your ability to bounce back from hard times. When you have a clear sense of what's meaningful to you, it's easier to be resilient. It's like having a light in the darkness. When you're facing a challenge, remembering what matters to you can give you the strength to overcome it.

For example, if you're passionate about your work, even on a bad day, that passion can motivate you to push through. Or, if family is your main focus, thinking of them can give you the power to stand back up after a fall.

Cultivating meaning in your life can start with reflecting on what truly matters to you. This could be your relationships, your career, hobbies, or even a personal cause. Once you identify these key areas, create your life around these things and think about them when you face hardship.

Like Friedrich Nietzsche said, "He who has a WHY to live can bear almost any how."

Before We Get Started…

Remember, mindfulness journaling is a personal practice, and these questions are meant to guide and inspire you. Feel free to adapt and modify them to suit your needs and preferences. Explore, reflect, and embrace the opportunity to deepen your self-awareness and cultivate a sense of inner peace.

Date ___ / ___ / ___ : S   M   T   W   Th   F   S

I feel: (please circle)

because _____ because _____ because _____ because _____ because _____

Today I Am Grateful For
1. _____
2. _____
3. _____

What could help transform today into a remarkable day?

Reflective Writing
How have my resilience and coping strategies evolved over the years?

_____

_____

_____

_____

_____

_____

_____

Which of the following is NOT a helpful coping strategy for managing stress?

a) Journaling
b) Procrastination
c) Exercise
d) Deep breathing

All Are Correct - Choose The Response You Feel Is Most Important To Remember

Date ___ / ___ / ___ : S M T W Th F S

I feel:
(please circle)

because _____ because _____ because _____ because _____ because _____

Today I Am Grateful For

1. _____
2. _____
3. _____

What could help transform today into a remarkable day?

Reflective Writing

What are the most effective resilience and coping strategies I can use to manage stress?

_____

_____

_____

_____

_____

_____

_____

Which of the following is a characteristic of resilient individuals?

a) Feeling overwhelmed easily
b) Accepting failure as permanent
c) Ignoring their emotions
d) Adapting to change

All Are Correct - Choose The Response You Feel Is Most Important
To Remember

Date ___ / ___ / ___ : S M T W Th F S

I feel:
(please circle)

because _____ because _____ because _____ because _____ because _____
_____ _____ _____ _____ _____

Today I Am Grateful For

1. _____
2. _____
3. _____

What could help transform today into a remarkable day?

Reflective Writing

Are there any negative coping strategies
I should avoid?

_____

_____

_____

_____

_____

_____

_____

Which of the following is an effective way to build resilience?

a) Avoiding all sources of stress
b) Overworking and pushing through challenges
c) Seeking support from others
d) Ignoring negative thoughts

All Are Correct - Choose The Response You Feel Is Most Important To Remember

Date ___ / ___ / ___ : S   M   T   W   Th   F   S

I feel:
(please circle)

because _____ because _____ because _____ because _____ because _____

Today I Am Grateful For

1. _____
2. _____
3. _____

What could help transform today into a remarkable day?

Reflective Writing

What are some useful strategies for building emotional resilience?

_____

_____

_____

_____

_____

_____

_____

Which of the following is a common way people cope with stress in unhealthy ways?

a) Talking to a friend about their feelings
b) Engaging in excessive exercise
c) Practicing mindfulness and meditation
d) Setting realistic goals and expectations

All Are Correct - Choose The Response You Feel Is Most Important To Remember

35

Date ___ / ___ / ___ : S   M   T   W   Th   F   S

I feel:
(please circle)

because because because because because
_____ _____ _____ _____ _____
_____ _____ _____ _____ _____

Today I Am Grateful For

1. _____
2. _____
3. _____

What could help transform today into a remarkable day?

Reflective Writing

How can I better prepare myself for the unexpected?

_____

_____

_____

_____

_____

_____

_____

_____

Which of the following is important for building resilience?

a) Avoiding challenges and difficult situations
b) Avoiding vulnerability and emotions
c) Developing a strong support system
d) Ignoring negative thoughts and feelings

All Are Correct - Choose The Response You Feel Is Most Important To Remember

Date ___ / ___ / ___ : S M T W Th F S

I feel:
(please circle)

because   because   because   because   because
_____   _____   _____   _____   _____
_____   _____   _____   _____   _____

Today I Am Grateful For

1. _____
2. _____
3. _____

What could help transform today into a remarkable day?

Reflective Writing

What are some ways I can help others to develop
their own resilience and coping strategies?

_____

_____

_____

_____

_____

_____

_____

Which of the following is NOT a potential benefit of practicing self-care?

a) Increased self-esteem
b) Improved physical health
c) Decreased resilience
d) Reduced stress and anxiety

All Are Correct - Choose The Response You Feel Is Most Important To Remember

Date ___ / ___ / ___ : S   M   T   W   Th   F   S

I feel:
(please circle)

because _____ because _____ because _____ because _____ because _____

Today I Am Grateful For

1. _____
2. _____
3. _____

What could help transform today into a remarkable day?

Reflective Writing

What are the most powerful tools I can use to cope with difficult situations?

_____

_____

_____

_____

_____

_____

_____

Which of the following is a helpful way to cope with failure and setbacks?

a) Blaming others
b) Giving up easily
c) Learning from mistakes
d) Ignoring the problem

All Are Correct - Choose The Response You Feel Is Most Important To Remember

41

Date ___ / ___ / ___ : S M T W Th F S

I feel:
(please circle)

because _____ _____
because _____ _____
because _____ _____
because _____ _____
because _____ _____

Today I Am Grateful For

1. _____
2. _____
3. _____

What could help transform today into a remarkable day?

Reflective Writing

How can I ensure I have enough emotional energy
to handle challenging times?

_____

_____

_____

_____

_____

_____

_____

Which of the following is a common barrier to building resilience?

a) A strong support system
b) Asking for help
c) Fear of failure
d) Practicing self-care

All Are Correct - Choose The Response You Feel Is Most Important To Remember

Date ___ / ___ / ___ : S M T W Th F S

I feel:
(please circle)

because _____ because _____ because _____ because _____ because _____
_____ _____ _____ _____ _____

Today I Am Grateful For

1. _____
2. _____
3. _____

What could help transform today into a remarkable day?

Reflective Writing

What are the most important skills needed to
build resilience?

_____

_____

_____

_____

_____

_____

_____

Which of the following is NOT a recommended way to manage overwhelming emotions?

a) Avoiding them
b) Talking to a trusted friend or family member
c) Expressing them through creative outlets
d) Practicing mindfulness and relaxation

All Are Correct - Choose The Response You Feel Is Most Important To Remember

Date ___ / ___ / ___ : S M T W Th F S

I feel:
(please circle)

because _____ because _____ because _____ because _____ because _____

Today I Am Grateful For

1. _____
2. _____
3. _____

What could help transform today into a remarkable day?

Reflective Writing

How can I ensure I stay mentally healthy during stressful times?

_____

_____

_____

_____

_____

_____

_____

Which of the following is NOT a helpful approach for problem-solving?

a) Avoidance
b) Break down the problem into smaller parts
c) Brainstorming solutions
d) Seeking guidance from others

All Are Correct - Choose The Response You Feel Is Most Important To Remember

Date ___ / ___ / ___ : S   M   T   W   Th   F   S

I feel:
(please circle)

because _____   because _____   because _____   because _____   because _____

Today I Am Grateful For

1. _____
2. _____
3. _____

What could help transform today into a remarkable day?

Reflective Writing

Are there any activities I can do to promote resilience and coping skills?

_____

_____

_____

_____

_____

_____

_____

Which of the following is a key component of self-compassion?

a) Negative self-talk
b) Self-criticism
c) Mindfulness
d) Kindness and understanding

All Are Correct - Choose The Response You Feel Is Most Important To Remember

Date ___ / ___ / ___ : S   M   T   W   Th   F   S

I feel:
(please circle)

because _____   because _____   because _____   because _____   because _____

Today I Am Grateful For

1. _____
2. _____
3. _____

What could help transform today into a remarkable day?

Reflective Writing
How can I remain focused on my goals during difficult times?

_____

_____

_____

_____

_____

_____

_____

Which of the following is NOT an example of resilience?

a) Giving up easily

b) Overcoming challenges

c) Seeking help when needed

d) Adapting to change

All Are Correct - Choose The Response You Feel Is Most Important To Remember

Date ___ / ___ / ___ : S   M   T   W   Th   F   S

I feel:
(please circle)

because   because   because   because   because
_____   _____   _____   _____   _____
_____   _____   _____   _____   _____

Today I Am Grateful For

1. _____
2. _____
3. _____

What could help transform today into a remarkable day?

Reflective Writing
What are the most effective ways to manage my
emotions in challenging situations?

_____

_____

_____

_____

_____

_____

_____

_____

Which of the following is a key aspect of a growth mindset?

a) Avoiding challenges
b) Dwelling on past mistakes
c) Embracing change
d) Giving up easily

All Are Correct - Choose The Response You Feel Is Most Important
To Remember

Date ___ / ___ / ___ : S M T W Th F S

I feel:
(please circle)

because because because because because
_____ _____ _____ _____ _____
_____ _____ _____ _____ _____

Today I Am Grateful For

1. _____
2. _____
3. _____

What could help transform today into a remarkable day?

Reflective Writing

How can I use my strengths to build
resilience and cope better?

_____

_____

_____

_____

_____

_____

_____

Which of the following is NOT a recommended way to cope with stress and anxiety?

a) Practicing self-compassion
b) Avoiding relaxation techniques
c) Setting realistic expectations
d) Engaging in physical activity

All Are Correct - Choose The Response You Feel Is Most Important To Remember

Date ___/___/___: S M T W Th F S

I feel:
(please circle)

because _____ because _____ because _____ because _____ because _____

Today I Am Grateful For

1. _____
2. _____
3. _____

What could help transform today into a remarkable day?

Reflective Writing

What are some strategies I can use to stay positive during difficult times?

_____

_____

_____

_____

_____

_____

_____

Which of the following is a helpful way to build resilience in the workplace?

a) Ignoring conflicts and challenges
b) Developing strong relationships with coworkers
c) Avoiding asking for help
d) Focusing solely on work and ignoring personal life

All Are Correct - Choose The Response You Feel Is Most Important To Remember

As we reach the final pages of this journey through "Positive Mindset," I want to extend my heartfelt thanks to you. Your commitment to exploring positivity and its transformative power is not only commendable but a testament to your desire for personal growth and a richer, more fulfilling life experience.

Remember, the journey towards a positive mindset is ongoing and ever-evolving. Each day presents new opportunities to apply these principles, to learn, and to grow. I encourage you to revisit these pages whenever you need a reminder of your incredible potential to foster positivity and resilience in the face of life's challenges.

As we part ways, I leave you with a quote that has been a guiding star in my journey: "The greatest discovery of any generation is that a human can alter his life by altering his attitude."

– William James.

Thank you for allowing me to be a part of your journey. May your path be filled with light, hope, and endless possibilities. Farewell, and may you carry the spirit of positivity with you, today and always.

With gratitude and best wishes,

Sensei Paul David

Reflective Writing

The End

As you close the pages of this mindfulness journal, remember that each word you've written is a step on your journey towards self-awareness and inner peace. Embrace the moments of clarity, the revelations, and even the uncertainties you've encountered along the way. Let this journal be a testament to your growth and a reminder that every day offers a new opportunity to be present, to observe, and to appreciate the simple wonders of life. Carry these lessons forward, and may your path be filled with mindful moments and serene reflections. Until we meet again in these pages, be gentle with yourself and stay anchored in the now.

Mindfulness isn't difficult, we just need to remember to do it.

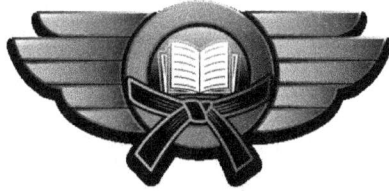

Thank You!

If you found this book helpful, I would be grateful if you would **post an honest review on Amazon** so this book can reach other supportive readers like you!

All you need to do is digitally flip to the back and leave your review. Or visit amazon.com/author/senseipauldavid click the correct book cover and click on the blue link next to the yellow stars that say, "customer reviews."

As always...
It's a great day to be alive!

Get/Share Your FREE SSD Mental Health Chronicles at
www.senseiselfdevelopment.care

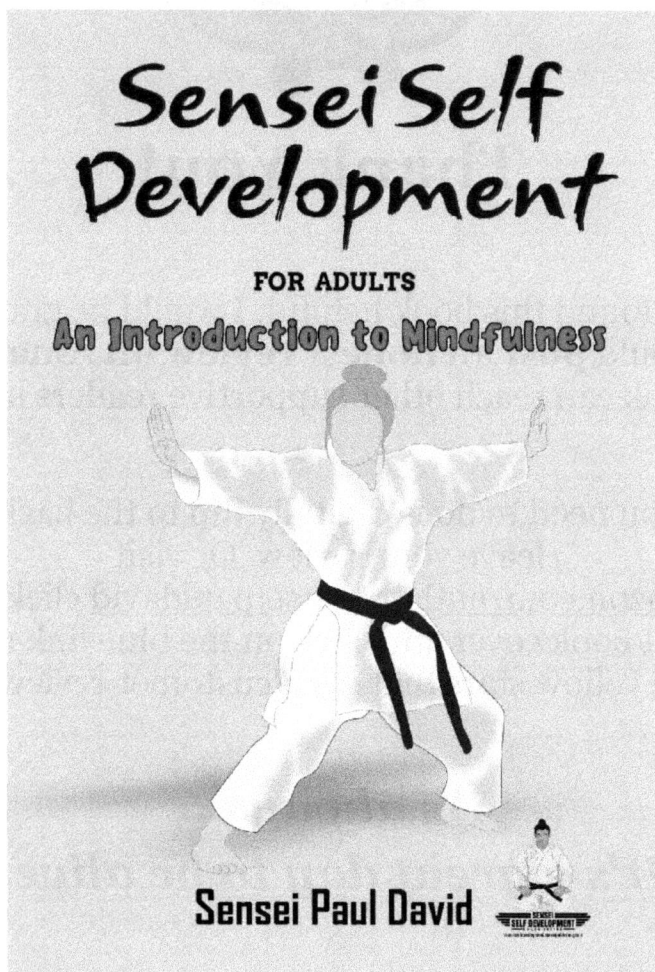

Sensei Self
Development

FOR ADULTS

An Introduction to Mindfulness

Sensei Paul David

Check Out The SSD Chronicles
Series CLICK HERE

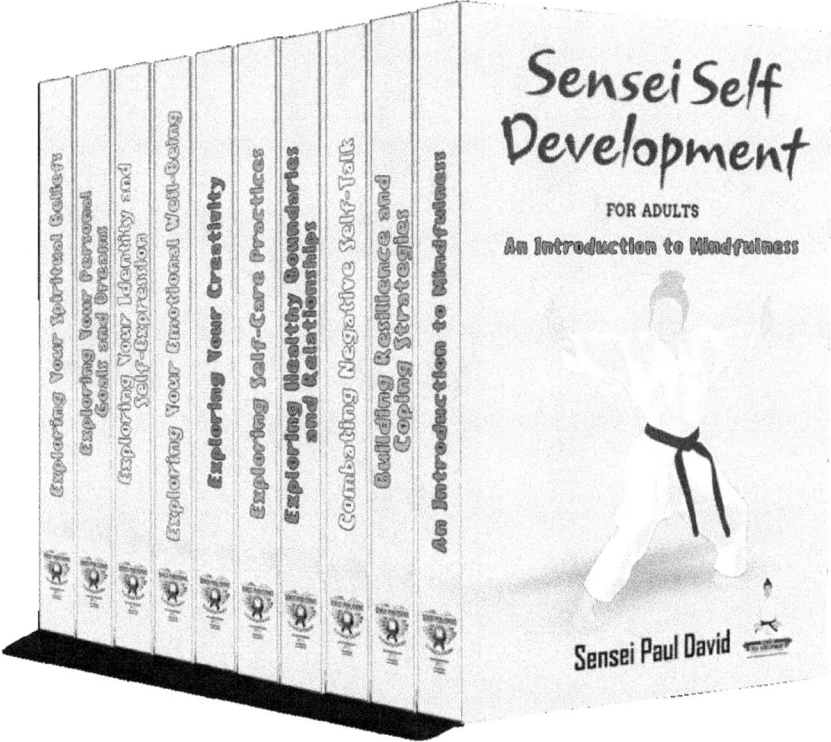

Get/Share Your FREE All-Ages Mental Health eBook Now at

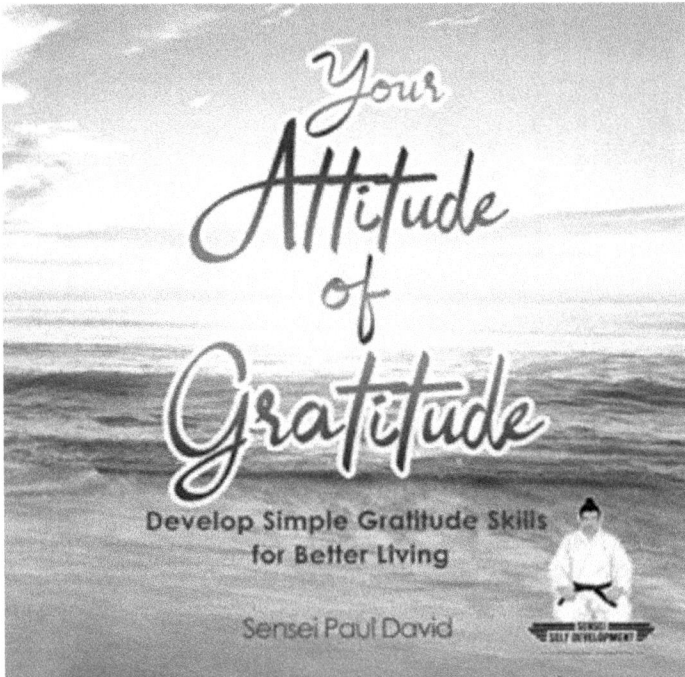

www.senseiselfdevelopment.com

Or CLICK HERE

Click Another Book In The SSD BOOK SERIES:

senseipublishing.com/SSD_SERIES

CLICK HERE

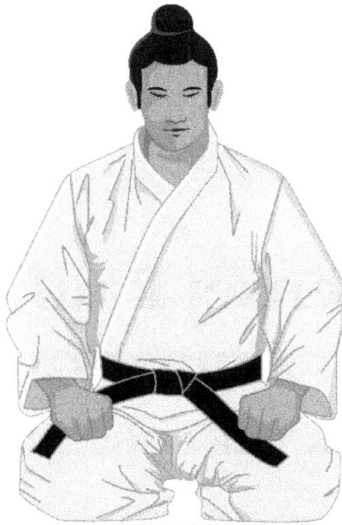

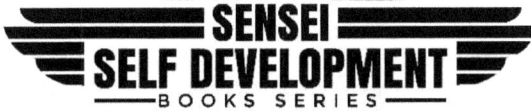

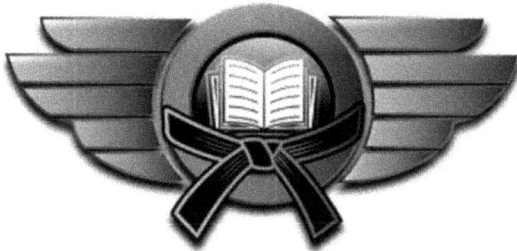

Join Our Publishing Journey!

If you would like to receive FREE BOOKS, please visit **www.senseipublishing.com**. Join our newsletter by entering your email address in the pop-up box

Follow Sensei Paul David on Amazon

CLICK THE LOGO BELOW

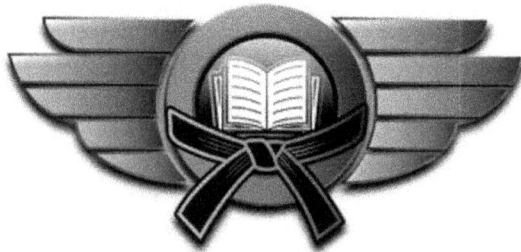

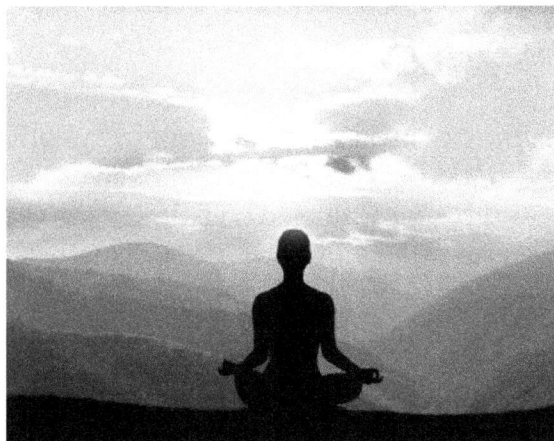

FREE BONUS!!!
Experience Over 25 FREE Engaging Guided
Meditations!

Prized Skills & Practices for Adults & Kids. Help
Restore Deep-Sleep, Lower Stress, Improve Posture,
Navigate Uncertainty & More.

Download the Free Insight Timer App and click the
link below:
http://insig.ht/sensei_paul

About Sensei Publishing

Sensei Publishing commits itself to helping people of all ages transform into better versions of themselves by providing high-quality and research-based self-development books with an emphasis on mental health and guided meditations. Sensei Publishing offers well-written e-books, audiobooks, paperbacks and online courses that simplify complicated but practical topics in line with its mission to inspire people towards positive transformation.

It's a great day to be alive!

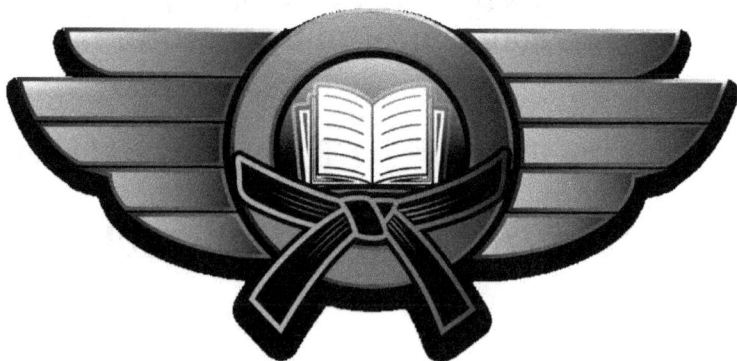

About the Author

I create simple & transformative eBooks & Guided Meditations for Adults & Children proven to help navigate uncertainty, solve niche problems & bring families closer together.

I'm a former finance project manager, private pilot, jiu-jitsu instructor, musician & former University of Toronto Fitness Trainer. I prefer a science-based approach to focus on these & other areas in my life to stay humble & hungry to evolve. I hope you enjoy my work and I'd love to hear your feedback.

- It's a great day to be alive!

Sensei Paul David

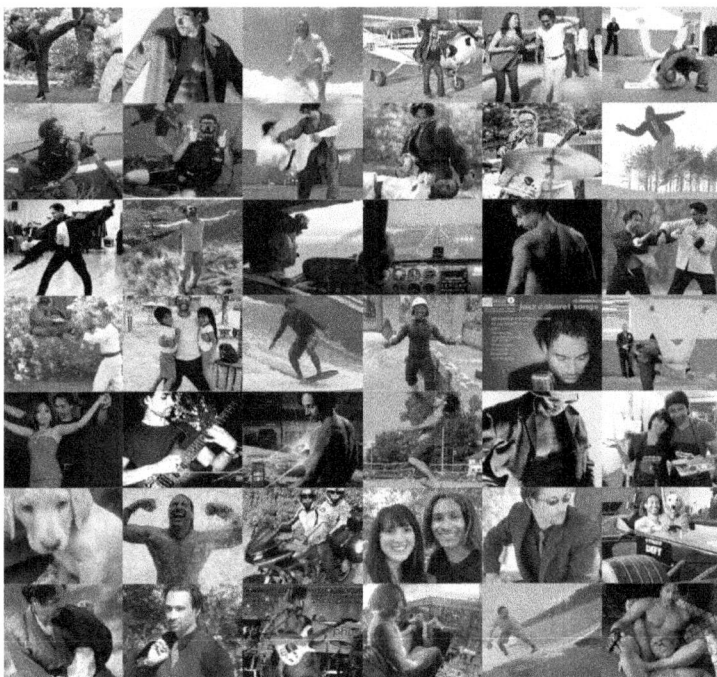

Scan & Follow/Like/Subscribe: Facebook, Instagram, YouTube: @senseipublishing

Scan using your phone/iPad camera for Social Media
Visit us at www.senseipublishing.com and sign up for our
newsletter to learn more about our exciting books and to
experience our FREE Guided Meditations for Kids & Adults.

A Message From The Author:
Sensei Paul David

Dear Reader,

Welcome to the world of mental health journaling – a sacred space for self-reflection, growth, and healing. Within these pages, you hold the power to uplift your spirit, invigorate your mind, and nourish your goals.

In a world that often moves at blink-and-you'll-miss-it speed, it's crucial to make time for self-care and self-discovery.

Anxiety, stress, and emotional turbulence may have clouded your mind, making it difficult to find clarity and peace within. But fear not! Together, we will navigate the labyrinth of emotions, and experiences, helping to simplify the path to mental well-being.

This journal is not merely a bunch of blank pages awaiting your words. It is your compassionate companion, offering solace and understanding during your unique journey. Here, you are free to unburden yourself, celebrate small and large victories, and confront the challenges that may still linger.

Join Our Publishing Journey!

If you would like to receive FUTURE FREE BOOKS and get to know us better, please click www.senseipublishing.com and join our newsletter by entering your email address in the pop-up box.

Follow Our Blog: senseipauldavid.ca

Follow/Like/Subscribe: Facebook, Instagram, YouTube:
@senseipublishing

Scan the QR Code with your phone or tablet

to follow us on social media: Like / Subscribe / Follow

Check Out Another Book In The
SSD BOOK SERIES:

senseipublishing.com/SSD_SERIES

CLICK HERE

SENSEI
SELF DEVELOPMENT
BOOKS SERIES

senseiselfdevelopment.senseipublishing.com

Get/Share Your FREE All-Ages Mental Health eBook Now at

www.senseiselfdevelopment.com

Or CLICK HERE

senseiselfdevelopment.com

_____

_____

If I don't finish 10 days of writing this journal, I
will promise to:

_____

_____

_____

_____

_____

_____

I will do the following things to ensure that I
write in my Sensei Self Development Journal
every day:

_____

_____

_____

_____

_____

_____

MY
COMMITMENT

I, _____

commit to writing This Sensei Self
Development Journal for at least 10 days in a
row, starting: _____

Writing this journal is valuable to me because:

_____

_____

_____

_____

_____

_____

If I finish a minimum of 10 consecutive days of
writing in this journal, I will reward myself by:

_____

_____

_____

_____